Intermittent Fasting for Beginners:

The Proven Way to Lose Weight, Build Muscle and Live a Healthy, Food-Stress-Free Lifestyle

By Jason Michaels

Table of Contents

for any hardship or damages that may befall them after undertaking information described herein.

Additionally, the information in the following pages is intended only for informational purposes and should thus be thought of as universal. As befitting its nature, it is presented without assurance regarding its prolonged validity or interim quality. Trademarks that are mentioned are done without written consent and can in no way be considered an endorsement from the trademark holder.

Disclaimer: Consult a physician before beginning any kind of diet or weight loss regime.

Do not follow these diets if you are pregnant, breastfeeding or suffer from diabetes.

Introduction

Congratulations on purchasing *"Intermittent Fasting for Beginners: The Proven Way to Lose Weight, Build Muscle and Live a Healthy Lifestyle."* Thank you for doing so.

The food pyramid model for eating was first introduced in Sweden in 1974 and spread throughout other Scandinavian countries, Sri Lanka and West Germany. The food pyramid was introduced to the United States in 1992 and was replaced by MyPlate in 2011 after people realized the pyramid was terribly erroneous. The model's focus on heavy carbohydrate intake contributed to making the citizens of the United States among the world's largest populations of obese people.

At the same time, the quick-paced, modern lifestyle also contributed to poor eating habits. Fast food, with its emphasis on cheap starchy and sugary food, replaced many healthy homemade meals.

According to the World Health Organization, as of 2014 more than 1.9 billion adults over the age of 18 were overweight worldwide, and 600 million of those would be considered obese. Additionally, 41 million children younger than 5 were considered overweight or obese.

However, a recent movement toward natural eating brought a resurgence in various popular diets and eating habits that resemble those of our ancestors. One of these diets involves the practice of intermittent fasting.

The following chapters describe what fasting is, the science behind fasting, and why meal timing is irrelevant. The various intermittent fasting structures are explained, as well as how to use intermittent fasting to lose weight or to build muscles. This book also gives specific information about meal plans, eating schedules, and exercising.

There are plenty of books on this subject on the market. Thanks again for choosing this one! Every effort was made to ensure it is full of as much useful information as possible. Good luck in your journey toward a thinner, healthier you!

Chapter 1: What is Fasting?

There are a number of different definitions as to how long between meals, or what intake determines a fast. Fasting can be summarized as the deliberate act of not eating or drinking for a period of time.

Sometimes a person drinks juice ("juice fasting") or water but does not eat. This can be considered a fast depending on your diet plan.

Technically, we all fast daily if we get eight hours of sleep every night. If we also don't eat several hours before bedtime, or if we skip breakfast, we have had a mini-fast of 12 hours. It's that easy.

"Intermittent fasting" is when a person skips at least one meal, then eats, then fasts, and so on. A person is considered to have entered a period of fasting if they have not eaten for more than eight hours.

Fasting is not a new phenomenon however. Humans have been fasting for thousands of years. Historically, people fasted for various reasons, not just limited to health. These included religious and medical reasons.

Fasting in History: Religious reasons

When fasting is done for religious reasons, it is sometimes viewed as a symbolic gesture that serves to teach people to not be selfish or act upon carnal desires. Various religions also consider fasting to aid in meditation. Thus, religious leaders often tell parishioners to engage in "fasting and prayer."

Buddhist monks and nuns fast daily after their noon meals until the next morning. They think of this practice as something that aids in meditation and contributes to good health, however, they do not consider this daily practice to be fasting. Buddhists consider long-term periods of eating very little food to be fasting by their traditional definition, and they fast in this sense when they want to practice intense meditation.

Many members of Christianity embrace the practice of fasting because of various Bible passages, such as Isaiah 58:6-7, which was written to the Israelites and spoke of an "acceptable fast." This had to do with following all commandments.

Fasting is practiced in some, but not all denominations of Christianity.

Those that do engage in this practice include both Pentecostals and Charismatics as the result of individual choice, but the Charismatics commonly choose to do it once weekly.

The Eastern Orthodox Church and the Catholic Church practice a forty-day partial fast every year. The Eastern Orthodox Church considers fasting as part of a connection between body and the soul. The Ethiopian Orthodox Church does not eat meat or consume milk in any form for several weeks, several times every year.

Roman Catholics have strict fasting rules for parishioners who are between the ages of 18 and 59 during Lent. The Anglican Church also has strict fasting rules, as do the Assyrian Church of the East. Lutheran and Reformed churches take a much less stringent position on fasting.

The Church of Jesus Christ of Latter Day Saints, better known as the Mormons fast two meals on the first Sunday of every month, and the money saved by not eating is donated to the church. Hindus fast on particular day of the month.

This historical practice demonstrates that the act of fasting is one that is more than just a passing health fad, and more so an act deep seated across societies worldwide.

Fasting for medical reasons

Patients are required to abstain from eating food before their blood, cholesterol, or glucose levels are tested and before they are screened for diabetes. That is because food can interfere with test results. A partial fast that only allows clear liquids to be consumed is required just before a colonoscopy.

Patients must not eat before having a major surgery that involves the use of anesthesia. If a patient eats just before surgery, he could vomit, inhale the vomit and die while he is unconscious. Regurgitation while under anesthesia is rare, however, so fasting may no longer be required of surgery patients in the near future.

Fasting for health reasons

There are several benefits of intermittent fasting over other weight loss methods.

Detoxification - One benefit is the fact that fasting causes the body to detoxify. Toxic buildup occurs because of a poor diet and because of eating frequently (meals eaten less than six hours apart). The body needs to take a break from processing food so that it can cleanse the digestive tract.

Weight Loss - When people fast, the body helps them lose weight in two ways. Most people carry between five and twenty pounds of food in their intestines. When a person fasts, their body gets rid of much of the impacted feces on its own, although drinking sea salt in warm water or senna tea while fasting helps tremendously. Old waste matter is one source of the extra weight.

Not including water retention, the other source of extra weight is, of course, fat. When the body does not receive food within about 12 hours, it starts to use stored-up fat for fuel.

Hunger Management - Another benefit of intermittent fasting is hunger management. When you are not fasting, your blood sugar level decreases and your brain receives a message that you are hungry. When you fast intermittently, however, your body burns the fat and the hunger hormones are turned off. This allows our bodies to reduce the feeling of hunger and we are less likely to be struck by food cravings that are prone to throw us off our diets.

Reduced Risk of Type II Diabetes - Since intermittent fasting causes your body to burn all of the glucose in your body before it burns fat for energy, your blood sugar levels remain low. Low blood sugar levels decrease the risk of getting Type II diabetes. A 2009 study published by the *Scandanvian Journal of Clinical and*

Laboratory Investigation found that intermittent fasting resulted in a 3 to 6% reduction of blood sugar that caused a 20 to 31% reduction in insulin. Intermittent fasting also increases the dieter's sensitivity to insulin.

Slowing Down of the Aging Process - The lowering of blood sugar that happens during intermittent fasting forces the body's cells to remove unhealthy mitochondria, which reduces production of free radicals. When there are less free radicals, there is less oxidative stress which leads to a slowing down of the aging process.

Reduced Risk of Cancer – Whether or not intermittent fasting reduces the risk of cancer is a topic that continues to be heavily debated, but it is thought to at least be effective against breast cancer. However, one study performed by USC's D. Valter Longo and reported in the research journal *Cell Metabolism* that was done on 10 cancer patients demonstrated that intermittent fasting caused the fasting patients to respond better to the chemotherapy and to have better cure rates than cancer patients who did not fast. Cancer results from uncontrolled growth of cells, and those cells rely on glucose to grow. That is why less food would logically slow down the growth of cancer cells.

Longevity – Cell Metabolism also reported on numerous studies on rats demonstrated that intermittent fasting caused the rats to live 83% longer than the rats that were fed regularly.

Other anecdoctal eveidence - Various conditions alleviated by fasting, including constipation, stomach problems, addictions, rheumatic conditions, arthritis, asthma, heart disease, high blood pressure, high cholesterol levels, poor pancreas performance, sleep problems, mood swings, and mild depression. People have reported experiencing an increase in energy, clarity of mind, an increase in sex drive, a feeling of being clean inside, and a sense of overall well-being after they fast.

Chapter 2: The Science Behind Intermittent Fasting

A General Understanding

When a person eats regularly, the body breaks down the food that is eaten into glucose. Glucose triggers the production of insulin. Insulin helps the body use the glucose for energy and stores the unused glucose as fat because the fat is not used for energy.

After 12 hours of fasting, the body starts to burn fat, the body is forced to burn the stored fat because there is no glucose left to use for fuel. This is when weight loss happens. This is also the most effective time to exercise.

As fasting is most often thought of as not consuming calories at all for a period of time. Intermittent fasting is fasting for a short while and then starting back up with eating, cycling back and forth between eating and not eating.

Ancient man hunted for food after he went without food for several hours. This was not by choice, he fasted intermittently on a daily basis due to a lack of consistent food supply (and convenience stores!). Intermittent fasting brought about optimum and constant burning of fat for fuel rather than glucose. This was compounded by consuming only natural, healthy food. The hard life they led forced them into a healthy way of eating.

General calorie restriction is undernourishment without malnourishment, so as long as a person is not undernourished for long periods of time and he eats quality food when he eats, his body does not suffer from any health based consequences.

Clinical Studies

Many studies have been done on the effects of calorie restriction (low-calorie diets) on the health of humans and animals, but the effects of intermittent fasting on humans where no food is allowed occasionally has not been widely clinically studied.

One study that was performed by Martin, Mattson and Maudsley (of the United States National Institutes of Health) in 2006 and reported by the journal *Aging Research Reviews* indicated that the effects of intermittent fasting on health are similar to those of low-calorie diets.

Both calorie restriction and intermittent fasting put stress on cells, which brings about resistance to metabolic and environmental stress without doing any harm.
Calorie restriction and intermittent fasting also increase insulin sensitivity and reduce glucose and insulin levels.

Intermittent fasting studies performed on animals by Mark Mattson, senior investigator for the National Institute on Aging, showed that the test subjects who were subjected to intermittent fasting experienced better learning abilities, memory, reduced oxidative stress, and showed improvement in diseases.

Studies performed on humans showed that the body goes to fat stores for energy after 10 to 16 hours of fasting. Not surprisingly, the studies also showed that the body starts to quickly bring down a person's weight when a person combines intermittent fasting with a low-calorie diet that consists of quality food.

Mattson thought that perhaps the body resists disease because fasting puts the body's cells under mild stress, which brings about adaptation from the stress. This is what the body does when a person exercises.

Chapter 3: Why Meal Timing is Irrelevant for Weight Loss & Muscle Gain

You will notice that the timing of the meals eaten in each of the various intermittent fasting diet plans is different from that of the others, and yet all of these intermittent fasting plans work. For example, one diet has you not eating for an entire 24 hours, while others have you eating every day, but within smaller windows of time.

Time of Day

The time of day that you eat meals is irrelevant due to two main factors.

First of all, you will restrict the overall calorie count for each week while you are fasting intermittently, which means that you will burn more calories than you consume, no matter what time of day that you eat or drink those calories. This is the first law of thermodynamics and the basic science behind all diets or weight loss plans.

Granted, if you eat earlier in the day, you have time to burn the glucose, but any time you burn more calories than you eat and drink, you lose weight. Any additional exercise will also burn calories.

Secondly, you will burn fat instead of glucose around the clock when you fast intermittently. The time of day that you eat will not change that fact either.

Other diet plans may have you timing your carbohydrate intake. With intermittent fasting, this is no longer an issue. So long as you are at a net calorie deficit at the end of the day/week, the timing of eating carbs is not a big issue to the intermittent faster. You could only have carbs just before you work out in the gym so that you would have energy during that time. Contrary to that would be a program like the warrior diet which allows you to eat some carbs late at night when you do all of your eating for the day. This diet is ideal for gaining muscle weight and tends to be favored by bodybuilders who fast intermittently.

Eating carbohydrates in the morning is the kind of thing that we are used to when we are eating on a regular 3 meals a day schedule. However, 3 square meals a day has only been the societal norm for the past 300 years. Beforehand most advanced societies ate once or two daily. In fact, Yale University professor and editor of Food: The History of Taste states "There is no biological reason for eating three meals a day."

If you eat bread, pasta, etc., and do not fast, of course, it would be wise to eat carbohydrates in the morning so that you would have all day to burn off the large amount of glucose that will form in your body. Otherwise, the insulin would make all of that glucose convert to fat if you did not burn the required calories.

People argue that those of us who skip breakfast are fatter than people who eat breakfast, yet there is no data to back up this claim. They also claim that muscles will fall off if one is following an IF protocol. But the human metabolism does not change that quickly, which studies in both intermittent fasting and general fasting have shown.

In fact, the metabolic rate rises abruptly during the first 72 hours that a person fasts, and it takes the body between three and four days before a fast or a strict partial fast negatively affects metabolism. The idea that skipping one meal here and there affects metabolism, therefore, is erroneous.

Meal Frequency

When it comes to weight loss, there is much literature regarding "stoking the metabolic fire" if you were to eat six times per day and that skipping just one meal per day would slow down your metabolism.

This concept came from a misunderstanding of dietary-induced thermogenesis (DIT), which deals with how many calories the body burns while digesting food.

In the studies that were conducted which led to this notion that people need to eat frequently, the subject's metabolism was increasing because people ate more food during the day, not because they ate frequently.

If the study participants eating six meals per day ate the same number of calories daily as people who ate only three times per day did, there would have been no difference in the DIT. For example, six meals of 300 calories is the same total caloric intake as three meals of 600 calories.

What the participants did, though, was to eat more calories when they ate six times daily. Eating more food to raise metabolism is like being excited to save $100 by spending $800. It looks good on paper - but in actual terms, it just doesn't make sense.

From a practical standpoint, a smaller person needing a lower calorie intake on a diet where several small meals are required throughout the day would literally be eating a couple of bites of things at every meal if he or she were to stay within their calorie limit. So more meals for small people often does not make much practical sense, this is especially true for females.

The number of times that you eat in a day does not matter when it comes to retaining lean muscle tissue either, just as long as the daily intake of protein is high. Meal frequency only negatively affects lean muscles if the meal frequency promotes food choices that offer inadequate level of proteins to maintain muscle mass which is about 0.8g per lb of muscle mass over the course of a day.

Not only are low-sugar protein shakes effective sources of protein that will enable you to keep or build muscles, but these shakes also fill you up quickly and are low-calorie.

Chapter 4: The Various Intermittent Fasting Structures

16/8 Method

Best for: **People who will frequently work out in a gym, building muscles and losing fat.**

Creator: **This method was formulated by personal trainer and nutritional expert, Martin Berkhan**

How it Works: This diet is very simple. The dieter fasts for 16 hours per day if a man (14 hours per day if you are a woman) and eats within the remaining hours.

It does not matter which hours of the day that you choose, but as with all IF protocols you would likely want to schedule your fasting time around your sleeping hours.

If you do not work a first-shift job, the suggested way to schedule these daily fasts is to start your fast just after you eat dinner, sleep, exercise throughout the morning, and break your fast (at "breakfast") after you have fasted the 16 or 14 hours.

You can eat more carbohydrates on the days that you work out than on the days that you don't work out. On days that you do not work out, you need to consume more dietary fat.

Protein intake should be high every day, but even that depends on the amount of body fat that you have, your general activity level, your gender, age, goals, etc. As with all diets, keep processed food intake to a minimum. Protein shakes that contain fruit and vegetables in addition to the protein powder are acceptable as meal replacements, as are protein meal replacement bars (though in moderation, as many of these contain high levels of sugar).

If you follow this schedule, the only time you might feel a little hungry would be in the morning. If you are not working out, drink water, black coffee, unsweetened tea, or green tea during these late hours in your fast. If you put lemon in your water, you will further suppress the hunger. The caffeine in both coffee and tea increase the intensity of the fat burning that is occurring during these hours in addition to suppressing hunger.

Green tea suppresses hunger, burns fat, and also increases your metabolism. It increases metabolism because it has various bioactive properties such as EGCG as well as the aforementioned caffeine. These agents also interact with your hormones to better break down the fat.

Using this plan, the most effective time to work out is on an empty stomach. Working out while you are hungry doesn't sound like an attractive plan, but there is a way to get around that. This answer is drinking BCAA protein shake just before you work out.

Assuming you are doing this in the morning, you can then break your fast by eating something. If you like to work out in the evening, schedule your workout one or two hours after you have eaten.

Pros: People find this diet attractive because the timing and the frequency of meals is fairly flexible on the days that you don't work out, although most people still break up their eating into three meals.

Cons: This diet has strict guidelines as to what food you can eat, especially when it comes to your workout days. Some people find it hard to stick to the program because of this inflexibility.

EatStopEat

Best for: People who already eat healthy and are just needing a little boost.

Creator: This method was created by Brad Pilon, who had a background in nutrition and in the sports supplement industry. He created it based on the fact that brief, regular fasts help people to lose weight while retaining muscle mass.

How it Works: On this diet, the dieter does not eat for 24 hours one or two days per week. He or she can have calorie-free drinks (no milk or sugar) during the fasting days and then eat as they normally eat during the other days.

The rationale is simply to cut out overall calories taken in, however, doing a small amount of resistance training during just three of the days that you eat is key to losing weight and improving your overall body composition. Just simple compound exercises focusing on full body training (squats, deadlifts, bench press) during those three days will make the difference. Exercising on days that you eat sets this plan apart from some of the other plans that require you to work out on an empty stomach.

Start this fast after dinner one day and break it at dinner the next day, having only skipped breakfast and lunch. If you are new to fasting, you should fast just one day per week in the beginning. In time, you can increase this to fast two days per week. If even one day proves to be too difficult, start with just a 15-hour fast and add another hour with each fast that you do. Start a fast on a day that you will be naturally busy or when you are not scheduled to eat with other people.

Some people schedule a fast just before they attend a party because they can break their fast eating the party food (in moderation) without feeling guilty. It is best to not eat any junk food. But if you will attend a party anyway, this is one way to not lose any ground where your weight is concerned.

Pros: This plan is flexible. If you can't go without food for 24 hours, you can start with just 15 hours and work your way up as your body adjusts to fasting. Another good thing about this diet is that you do not count calories, weigh food, or restrict your diet (other than avoiding a free-for-all, junk food diet). Also, this diet retains lean muscle tissue better than the other methods do.

Cons: People can suffer headaches, fatigue, foul moods, or anxiety when they suddenly go without food for 24 hours. People also tend to binge-eat when they come off of this fast, finding self-control hard when they are hungry.

The Warrior Diet

Best for: Disciplined, devoted people who can follow rules.

Creator: This plan was formulated by fitness expert, Ori Hofmekler, who studied how the lean and muscular ancient Romans and Spartans ate.

How it Works: The ancient Roman and Spartan armies ate very little during the day and then feasted on food they hunted during the evenings. If body building is your thing, this should be your intermittent fasting diet of choice.

This diet is similar to the Martin Berghan's diet except you eat very small portions of food for 20 hours every day and then eat a lot of food during a period of just four hours every evening.

Even this diet needs to be eased into because the dieter can experience the same symptoms of hunger as if they didn't eat anything at all for all of those hours.

In your first week, skip breakfast once or twice a week. Skip breakfast three or four times the next week. Move into skipping lunch and work on up to skipping all breakfasts and lunches every day.

You may nibble on raw fruits and vegetables, eat small amounts of protein, and drink fresh juice during the days. This maximizes the "fight or flight" response from the sympathetic nervous system. This response promotes alertness, boosts energy, and burns fat.

When you break your fast at night, you must eat particular food groups in a particular order. First, you eat broth, then vegetables, protein/meat, and then fat. You can eat carbohydrates at the end of your four-hour feasting period if you are still hungry.

Eating at night maximizes the parasympathetic nervous system, which helps the body to recuperate, become calm, relax, digest while the body uses the nutrients for growth and for repair. It may also help the body to produce fat-burning hormones that work on your fat the next day.

Another aspect of this diet is to do strength training during the daytime. Do squats, pull-ups, high jumps, press-ups, frog jumps and sprints. Select three of these activities, doing two sets of five minutes each during a thirty-minute period of time that you set aside every day. Drink a protein shake before you exercise.

Pros: A person who can regularly follow this diet will turn his or her body into a fat-burning and muscle-forming machine! One also gets to eat something during the fasting time, which helps the person endure the fasting hours. People experience increased energy and greater loss of fat when they adopt this eating style.

Cons: The strict schedule and eating guidelines are hard for some people to follow, especially if they have to attend a lot of social gatherings. Additionally, some people prefer to not eat large meals late at night.

Alternate Day Fasting

Best for: Disciplined people who have a weight goal in mind.

Creator: This diet was formulated by Dr. James Johnson especially for goal-minded disciplined dieters.

How it Works: Of the two intermittent fasting diets that mainly have weight loss in mind, this one is better optimized for your end goal.

On this diet, the dieter does a partial fast every other day, eating a limited amount of food for one day and then a normal amount the next day, and so on.

Because there are seven days in the week and the diet follows a schedule by the week day, the dieter uses three specific days of every week to do a partial fast. Dieters using this model commonly choose to diet on Mondays, Wednesdays, and Fridays.

On those days, the dieter consumes only one-fifth of the normal number of calories that he or she consumes on the other days. If you are a man, you likely take in about 2,500 calories per day. If you are a woman, you likely consume about 2,000 calories per day. Therefore, you would consume 500 or 400 calories on Mondays, Wednesdays, and Fridays, which can easily be done by drinking protein shakes.

Protein shakes are very filling and are also low in calories. High-protein foods and vegetables will also help you to fill up faster. The experts sometimes recommend protein shakes for just the first two weeks of the diet and real food from the third week onward.

Working out is not advised on this program, If you must work out while on this diet, do a lighter version of your regular workouts on the days that you eat normally.

Pros: This diet can effectively drop about 2.5 pounds of weight per week for dieters who cut their calorie intake between 20 and 35 percent, and this is done without the dieter feeling hungry or having to follow a difficult schedule. Additionally, dieting on alternate days never allows leptin levels to fall, which means that the body never stops losing the fat.

Cons: The dieter must be careful to not binge eat on their off days. This is not a program aimed for beginners or those who only need a slight reduction in weight.

The 5:2 Diet

Best for: People who are not sensitive to blood sugar levels.

Creator: This diet became popular because of the work of Dr. Michael Mosley, who was also a journalist.

How it Works: In this diet, you eat normally for five days of the week and reduce your calorie intake for two days of the week that are not consecutive days. Decide on the two days of the week you will diet and diet on those days every week.

When you eat normally, the calorie count needs to be 2,500 for men and 2,000 for women. On the partial fasting days, your calories should be 600 for men and 500 for women. You also consume those calories in two meals on fasting days, with 300 calories per meal for men and 250 calories per meal for women.

Green smoothies made of zucchini, celery, broccoli, lentils, kales, collards, mustard, and spinach are low in calories and will fill you up fast. Watermelon and broth-based soups will also fill you up fast. Drink a lot of water on the partial fasting days.

Pros: The plan is easy. It is similar to the EatStopEat plan, but you fast (partially) just two days of the week.

Cons: This diet is not advisable for people who have a history of eating disorders, or are sensitive to fluctuations in blood sugar levels.

Chapter 5: Intermittent Fasting for Weight Loss

As you read in the previous chapter, programs exist for people whose goal is to lose the fat and not necessarily to build up muscle.

If weight loss is your main goal, you have a choice between the Alternate Day Fast or the 5:2 Diet if using intermittent fasting.

Alternate Day Fast	The 5:2 Diet
Fasting schedule	
Partially fast three full alternate days.	Partially fast two full alternate days.

Fasting time food/cal

Men=500; Wm=400	Men=600; Wm=500
Vegetable soup, salad or other veggies with chicken or turkey, eggs	Green (veggie based) smoothies,

Divide calories between two meals with veggies, and yogurt with berries being good options

Eat time food/cal

Men=2,500; Wm=2,000	Men=2,500; Wm=2,000
Normal food, little junk.	Normal food, little junk.

Missed meals

N/A	N/A

Exercise

None

None to very light

Restrictions

None

Glucose-sensitive
people

Pros

Effective; no hunger

Easiest; no hunger

Cons

Temptation to binge people

Not avail. to all

Chapter 6: Intermittent Fasting for Muscle Gain

If you want to gain muscle as you lose the fat, you can choose from the Leangains, EatStopEat, and the Warrior intermittent fasting plans.

16/8 (Berghan)	EatStopEat	Warrior
Fasting sched.		
Fast 16 hours daily. Many people start right after dinner to take advantage of sleep hours	Full fast 24 hours one or two days weekly. Many people start right after dinner. The next meal is dinner the next day. If	Fast 20 hours daily. Eating nightly. You will likely need to fast fewer hours when you start this diet and work up to 20 hours. This

	you cannot fast 24 hours. Begin with 15 hours and increase as required.	diet tells you to eat at night, so start your fast after your large dinner.
Fast'g time food		
No calories except 10g BCAAs before a workout and 10g after a workout. Can drink unlimited water, black coffee and green tea	No calories. Can drink unlimited water, black coffee and green tea	Snack on small amounts of raw fruit and veggies or lean protein. Can drink unlimited water, black coffee and green tea

Eat time food		
Your regular diet with limited junk food. Everything in moderation. Eat more carbs on days you exercise and more fat on your off days.	Your regular diet with limited junk food. Everything in moderation.	Eat food in this order: Broth, veggies, meat, additional carbs
Missed Meals		
One per day	Two per day	Two main meals (partial fast)

Exercise		
3-4 Days per week focusing on compound exercises. For fat burning, exercise in the mornings on an empty stomach with 10g BCAAS	3 Days Per week. Perform 3 of the following exercises: Squats, Leg extensions, dumbell lunges, seated calf raises, barbell or dumbell rows, pull-ups, bench press, incline press, barbell bicep curl, front dumbell raises	3-5 Days Per Week. Bodyweight Strength training consisting of squats, pull-ups, push-ups, high jumps, sprints, frog jumps for 30 minutes daily. Choose 3 exercises and perform 2 sets for 5 minutes each.

Restrictions		
None	None	None

Pros		
Flexible dieting and meal frequency	Flexible number of fasting hours. No calorie counting. No weighing food. No strict dieting restrictions. Retains lean muscles better than other programs	Prime your body to be a lean-muscle building and fat burning machine. Some snacking allowed outside of eating hours.

Cons		
Strict dietary guidelines, especially on fasting days, are hard for some people to follow	Long fasting times can cause mood swings, fatigue and headaches in some people.	Strict eating protocol can be difficult for some people to follow. Not ideal if you do not enjoy or prefer large meals - especially late at night

Chapter 7: Intermittent Fasting and Exercise

Food is the fuel that your body uses to power itself and to build new muscle when exercising. With that in mind, it shouldn't be surprising that the timing of your meals can easily have a serious impact both on how easily you will find a given workout and also how effective that workout will be.

Adding exercise to an intermittent fasting plan

It doesn't matter if you are training for endurance or training to improve your strength, your body primarily uses the glycogen found in stored carbohydrates to fuel your exercise. However, when your glycogen reserves are running low, such as when you are in the latter half of a period of fasting, then your body is going to need to look to other energy sources like fat to power your exercise routine. This means that you are likely to burn up to 20 percent more fat if you exercise during a fast as opposed to just after you have broken one.

Unfortunately, it is not all good news as when glycogen is in short supply in your body, you are also more likely to burn protein as well as fat. As protein is what helps to build muscles, exercising in the midst of fast is likely to cause you to lose muscle mass as well. Depending on how much you plan on exercising and how long it has been since you have eaten any carbs, your body may start burning protein for energy as soon as you get started.

This won't just affect how much you can bench press or how toned your body looks, it will also slow your metabolism which will make it more difficult for you to lose weight in the long run as your body naturally adapts to the number of calories you are consuming on a regular basis over time. As such, once your body gets used to the fact that you are consuming fewer calories per day on average your body will eventually get used to burning fewer calories each day to ensure that you have enough energy left over for the basics such as staying healthy, breathing and even staying upright throughout the day. It will typically take about a month of regular rounds of fasting for your body to adapt to the change.

Finally, when planning on how to merge your exercise plan with an intermittent fasting lifestyle it is important to keep in mind that it is naturally going to be more difficult to exercise on an empty stomach. When your blood sugar and glycogen levels are low you are going to naturally feel weaker than you otherwise would. What's more, if you don't schedule your workouts at the end of a fast then your results will suffer as your body won't have the tools it needs to build muscle.

Intermittent fasting and exercise tips

Prioritize low-intensity cardio: If you plan on exercising regularly while you are fasting, it is important to limit your cardio to low-intensity options. This means you should still be able to carry on a conversation with relative ease if you are exercising during a fast. Ideally, you are going to want to stick to things like a light jog or 25 minutes on a cardio machine and be sure not to push yourself too hard. It will also be extra important to listen to your body and take a breather if you start to feel dizzy or light-headed which is going to happen much more often than it otherwise would. If you ignore this advice and push your exercise intensity level to the limit then it will make the rest of your workout feel like much more of a struggle regardless of what you are doing.

Choose your battles: This is not to say that you should never push your body to the limit while fasting. Instead, it is important to time your more intense periods of exercise to about an hour after you have eaten. This will give your body time to process the nutrients you have provided for it and will help you to maximize the amount of fat you can lose while still staying properly fueled for the workout by having plenty of glycogen in your system which will also help to reduce the risk of low blood sugar levels. Additionally, if you can afford to alter your fasting schedule slightly, following up a high-intensity workout with a snack that is high in carbs is also encouraged because your muscles will have burned through the available glycogen while still being hungry for more.

Up your protein intake: Standard workout convention suggest that you are going to want to take in between 20 and 30 grams of protein every four hours while you are awake. While intermittent fasting makes this unattainable, you're should still aim to take in between 80 and 120 grams of protein per day. If you are planning a serious strength workout then you should plan to do so between two snacks, if not two full meals.

Additionally, it is important to keep in mind that snacks are going to be your friend, as long as your intermittent fasting plan supports them, of course. A snack or a meal consumed between 3 and 4 hours before a workout should be enough to keep your blood sugar up through a standard workout, or between 1 and 2 hours if you are prone to low blood sugar. These meals should include blood-sugar stabilizing protein along with fast-acting carbs, for example two pieces of whole wheat toast with banana slices and peanut butter. Additionally, sometime in the two hours after your workout you are going to want to try and consume approximately 20 grams of protein and 20 grams of carbs to ensure maximum muscle growth and to get your glycogen stores up high enough that you maintain energy until it is time to eat again.

Plan out your meals in the right way: Ideally you will want to be sure to consume a majority of your daily caloric intake in the period immediately following your workout period. This will not only make it easier for your body to generate lean muscle mass it will also make it easier to recover from the workout. In order to do this, you should start by determining the caloric requirements your body needs in order to build muscle.

To do so, you are going to need to determine your basal metabolic rate (BMR) which is the number of calories you burn while resting. The more lean muscle mass you have, the higher your BMR is going to be. Essentially what this means is that the more muscular physique you have, the more calories you are going to be burning around the clock.

The average human body burns about 60 percent of its daily calorie consumption just through natural daily processes. From there, the body burns about 30 percent of its energy on physical activity and 10 percent on digestion.

To determine how many calories your body burns while resting, you can use the following formula. First you will need to determine your weight in kilograms by dividing your current weight in pounds by 2.2. You will also need to determine your height in centimeters which can be found by taking your height in inches and multiplying by 2.54.

For men, your BMR will be equal to 66.47+(13.75 x weight in kilograms) + (5 x height in centimeters) – (6.75 x age).

For women, your BMR is going to be equal to (65.09 + (9.56 x weight in kilograms) + (1.84 x height in centimeters) – (4.67 x Age).

The end result is the number of calories you burn while your body is at rest. For example, for a man who weighs 200 lbs. their BMR would be about 2,200 calories. From there, you can use the Sterling-Pasmore Equation to determine how many calories you need based on your current amount of lean body mass. Each pound of lean muscle mass requires 13.8 calories to support it. You can determine your current lean body mass from standard body fat measurements.

Calculate lean muscle mass vs. fat mass:
Body fat % x scale weight= fat mass
Scale weight - fat mass= lean body mass

Once you have determined your BMR, you will want to account for the additional calories that are burned through exercise.

- If you live a primarily sedimentary lifestyle you will want to multiply your BMR by 1.2.

- If you perform a light exercise routine 3 or 4 times per week you you will want to multiply your BMR by 1.375.

- If you perform moderate exercise between 3 and 5 days per week you will want to multiply your BMR by 1.55

- If you exercise at a moderate intensity 6 or 7 days a week you will want to multiply your BMR by 1.725.

- If you are extremely active and exercise 6 or 7 days a week for 90 minutes or more you will want to multiply your BMR by 1.9 (this category is reserved for endurance athletes)

If you are not sure about your activity level, underestimate it rather than overestimate. Overestimating your activity levels can lead to excess calorie intake.

With your BMR in mind, you are then going to want to consume about 20 percent of those calories before you exercise for the best results. This meal or snack should be a quality mix of both carbs and protein. Then, when you are finished exercising you are going to want to consume about 60 percent of your total calories sometime in the next 2 to 4 hours. This might seem like a lot but if you focus on calorie dense foods it should not be a problem.

Additionally, with this type of setup it is important to keep in mind that you are typically better off focusing on a diet with more carbs and less fat to support muscle growth. This is due to the fact that, following a workout, you should focus on carb intake, instead of fats which can be detrimental. This doesn't mean you should eliminate all fats, it just means you are going to want to limit the number of fats you consume in your post-workout meals.

If you lead a mostly sedimentary lifestyle then you will want to take in about 31 calories per kilogram per day to maintain your weight. If you are a recreational athlete then this number will be between 33 and 38 calories. If you are an endurance athlete then this number will be between 35 and 50 calories based on your training. If you are strength training and exercising heavily then this will be between 30 and 60 calories based on your training.

If you are looking to build muscle mass then you should aim to ensure that you take in an additional 250 to 500 calories per day depending on the type of exercise you are doing. On the other hand, if you are exercising on a daily basis and are looking to lose weight then you should subtract an additional 300 calories from your daily intake. This will help you to not only lose weight, but also to maintain muscle mass in the process.

Specific exercise plans

Note: If you prefer to watch video demonstrations of certain exercises - many can be found on YouTube and on bodybuilding.com

Strength Protocol 1*:* In this plan, you normally fast through the evening, the night and the morning. After you are *twelve hours into your fast*, exercise for one hour.

There are four primary exercises that you do during this workout. They are weighted chin ups, bench press, squat, and deadlift. Don't over complicate things by adding other types of exercises.

Weighted chin ups – Start with pulldowns, chins and then weighted chins, depending on your relative strength. Start loading with five to ten pounds after you are able to do eight body weight repetitions. Stay between four and six reps.

Chins are considered better than pull-ups. Close-grip chins are also beneficial. You can focus on weighted chins and close-grip chins if you want to build up your biceps.

Bench press – You bench press to build up your chest, shoulders and triceps. If you struggle with bench press as a lot of beginners do, you can do dumbbell presses or weighted dips as a substitute exercise. Barbell exercises such as bench press have the advantage of allowing you to progress with smaller weight jumps, though. You can also incorporate secondary shoulder movements such as overhead press or overhead dumbbell press, however these should be kept to a maximum of 3 working sets per workout.

Squats – The single best lower body muscle building exercise. In order to execute a proper squat, you should keep your trunk upright, your spine in a neutral position and your shoulders relaxed. You will also want to point your toes outward while setting your feet at hip width.

From there, you will want to slowly lower your body down as you start the squat with the hips before following through with your knees. It is important to keep your core tight throughout this process, by taking a breath and holding it as you push your belly button backwards. This will help to protect your spine and create increased stability for your lower back.

It is also important to ensure the weight ends up being placed on your heels by driving your hips in behind you. While lowering yourself it is important to ensure your knees remain lined up with your big toe and that you do everything you can to ensure your knees don't buckle inward. Continue this motion until your hips are parallel to the floor before pushing up with your heels and returning to the starting position. Once there, you will want to exhale.

Squatting barefoot or in flat soled shoes (such as Converse sneakers) helps you maintain better form as regular running shoes have angled soles which can shift your weight forward.

Deadlift – Start by standing with your midfoot beneath the bar and stand so your hips are slightly more narrowed than when doing a squat. Point your toes so they are pointed slightly outward. Bend over without bending your legs to grab the bar. Grip it so your arms are about shoulder length apart. Your arms should be vertical when seen from the front. Drop into position through a knee bend and ensure you are low enough for your shins to touch the bar, taking special care to ensure the bar doesn't leave your midfoot. With a firm grip, straighten your back by raising your chest. Do this without changing position and ensuring the bar remains above your foot the entire time. Take a deep breath prior to standing up with the weight. The bar should maintain contact with your legs as you do so.

Return the weight to the floor by focusing on unlocking your knees and hips first. Lower the bar by moving your hips backward and keeping your legs straight. After the bar passes your knees, bend your legs even more. The bar should land on the ground directly over your midfoot

Note: With compound exercises like these, be sure to take appropriate rest between of three to five minutes between sets. When your strength improves, your muscles build. Either do a conditioning session or a strength session, but don't do both in the same session or else you will become only mediocre at both. Change parameters from week to week. Keep a training log and go for PRs on a regular basis.

Strength Protocol 2*: Do three sets for ten reps for four of the following exercises:

Leg extensions: For this exercise, you are going to need to use a leg extension machine. As you exhale, you are going to want to flex your quadriceps and extend your leg to its maximum length. Once your leg is fully extended you are going to want to lower the weight back to its original position slowly so that you remain in control, inhaling as you do so. It is important that you do not go past a 90-degree angle. Repeat as needed.

Dumbbell lunges: Hold a dumbbell in each hand so your arms hang naturally at your sides. Stand upright, holding your torso erect, and step forward with your dominant leg about 2 feet while your other leg in its original spot. Lower your body down until the knee of your back leg touches the ground, moving slowly to maintain your balance. Return to a standing position and repeat with both legs.

Seated calf raises: This exercise requires a machine. Start by sitting on the machine with your towns on the lower platform with your heels from it. Place your thighs beneath the leer pad before placing your hands atop the pad to prevent slippage. Breath in as you slowly lower your heels by bending your ankles until your calves reach full extension. Raise your heels and extend your ankles as high as they will go before contracting your calves and releasing your breath. Hold this position for a few seconds and repeat as needed.

Seated rows: To do this exercise you need a low pulley row machine that comes equipped with a V bar. Sit down at the machine in such a way that your knees are bent slightly and are not locked. Grab hold of the V bar utilizing a neutral grip where the palms of your hands face one another. Fully extend your arms and pull back until your torso reaches a 90-degree angle from your legs. You will want to ensure that your back is lightly arched and your chest is sticking out. Keep your torso stationary and pull the handles towards your torso while at the same time keep your arms close to it until you come into contact with your abs, breathing out while you do so and contracting your back muscles. Hold for a moment and then return to the starting position.

Pull-ups: Grip the bar with your arms extended to about shoulder-width and your palms facing down. Bend your knees so that you are hanging with your feet off of the floor and your arms straight. Pull yourself up by drawing your elbows towards the floor while keeping them close as well. Continue pulling until your chin is above the bar. Lower yourself in a controlled manner back towards the ground. Take a breath and repeat.

One-arm dumbbell preacher curl: Hold a dumbbell in one hand at arm's length and place your arm on top of an incline bench. While breathing in, lower the dumbbell by extending your upper arm completely. While exhaling, make use of your bicep to return the dumbbell to shoulder height. To ensure a full rep, make sure to bring your small finger higher than your thumb. Squeeze for 1 second in this position and return the dumbbell slowly to the starting position. Switch arms between each repetition.

Barbell bench press-wide grip: On a flat bench, lie back in such a way that your feet are firm on the floor. Take a wide grip on the bar with your palms facing forwards with a grip that is slightly less than shoulder width. Lift the bar and hold it with your arms locked above your head so the bar is perpendicular to the floor. Lower the bar to your chest slowly while breathing in. Hold the bar in place for 1 second before exhaling and returning the bar to the starting position, contracting your chest muscles as you do so. Ensure that it takes twice as long to bring the bar to your chest as it does to return it to the starting position.

Pushups with feet elevated: Lie on the floor facing down and place your hands at slightly-greater than shoulder width. Place your toes on an elevated flat surface. The greater the height of the flat surface, the more resistance you will find in the exercise. Using just your arms, lower yourself downwards until your chest is almost touching the floor, inhaling while you do so. Flex your pectoral muscles and return your body to the starting position, exhaling while you do so. Pause for a moment and then repeat.

Front dumbbell raises: Pick up two dumbbells, one in each hand, and stand straight with the weights on your thighs at arm's length. They should be gripped so that your palms are facing your thighs. Keep your torso stationary while lifting one of the dumbbells in a forward motion using a slight bend of the elbow. Continue until your arm is slightly north of parallel to the ground, exhaling as you do so. Inhale as you lower the dumbbell back to the starting position before repeating with the dumbbell held in the other arm. For additional resistance you can attempt both arms at the same time.

Strength Protocol 3: Strength train for 30 minutes. Do two sets for five reptitions each of three of the following exercises:

Squats: See above.

Pull-ups: See above.

Elevated push-ups: See above.

Then follow up with 2 of these 3 exercises until your allotted time has expired.

Jump squat: Holding a pair of dumbbells in such a way that your palms face one another. Lower yourself into a squat position before launching yourself into the air with as much force as you can muster. Take care to land softly with your knees bent. Stand before returning to the starting position and repeat as needed.

Sprints: After a brief warmup, run 10, 200-meter intervals with of a goal of making each in less than 36 seconds. Rest for 30 seconds between intervals. Decrease resting time as you improve.

Frog jumps: With your hands behind your head, squat from a standing position so that your head is facing straight ahead and your torso is straight. Jump forward, focusing on distance instead of height. Absorb the impact with your legs as your feet come into contact with the ground. Repeat for 1 minute before resting for 15 seconds.

Chapter 8: Different Intermittent Fasting Daily Schedules

16/8

Number of fasting days – You diet for 7 days per week, partially fasting. Note: It is actually a full fast except for the BCAA protein shake in the morning when you exercise.

Meal schedule – You start this diet right after dinner and do a partial fast for 16 hours. For example, you may finish your dinner at 8pm, sleep for the night, skip breakfast (except for the three times that you get 10 grams of protein) and then eat lunch at noon.

Fasting day calories – Every day is a partial fasting day on this diet. There is no calorie counting to do on this diet, but you do measure out the 10 grams of protein that you get three times every morning.

5 days off/2 days on

Number of fasting days – You diet for one or two days per week.

Meal schedule – You completely stop eating for 24 hours on your fasting day(s). People commonly fast for fewer hours than 24 when they first start this diet.

You can start this diet by fasting only 15 hours for one day a week. Fast for 16 hours the next week. Add one more hour of fasting the next week and keep adding an hour every week until you can go without food for 24 hours for one day a week. Fast for 15 hours on a second, but non-consecutive, day of the week and work up to 24 hours of fasting on that second day.

Start your fasts after dinner. Skip breakfast and lunch the next day. Then break the fast with dinner the next day.

Fasting day calories – This is a full fast with no calories consumed at all on these days. Black coffee, water and unsweetened green tea are acceptable.

20/4

Number of fasting days – You diet for 7 days per week, partially fasting.

Meal schedule – You partially fast for 20 hours, starting after a late-night dinner. You nibble during the day and feast on all food groups late at night during a four-hour window.

Fasting day calories – You do not count calories on this diet.

Alternate Day Fasting

Number of fasting days – You diet for 3 non-consecutive days per week, partially fasting. People usually choose Monday, Wednesday, and Friday to fast while on this plan, leaving the two consecutive weekend days as normal eating days.

Meal schedule - There are no rules on this diet as far as the number of meals go or the time that you eat is concerned.

Fasting day calories - Consume 500 calories if you are a man and 400 calories if you are a woman on your partial fasting days.

The 5:2 Diet

Number of fasting days – You diet for 2 non-consecutive days per week, partially fasting. Pick any two days of the week and try to stick with those days every week.

Meal schedule – Divide your allotted calories between two meals on the days that you fast.

Fasting day calories – Consume 600 calories if you are a man and 500 calories if you are a woman on your partial fasting days.

Building A Successful Fasting Mindset

While each type of intermittent fasting is beneficial in its own way, they can all feel both complicated and difficult to stick with if you don't approach them with the proper mindset. The following suggestions will make the process much easier to manage.

Be true to yourself: Just because intermittent fasting has the possibility to offer you the type of healthy lifestyle you are looking for, this in no way means that it is going to be compatible with your personality, habits and schedule. While you will likely be able to make it through a handful of fasts without giving in to the temptation to break them early, while doing so it is important to consider how difficult it was for you to follow through on, what your general relationship with food is like and what your natural eating patterns are. It is also important to keep in mind that intermittent fasting is a lifestyle, not a diet you are going to stick with for a short period of time and then discard.

As such, it is important that you take the time to have a conversation with yourself and determine if the internal and external factors that affect you ever day are going to align in such a way that fasting regularly is a realistic proposition. Regardless of what you ultimately decide, it is important to make the decision relatively early on as changing your eating patterns too regularly can have negative consequences for your body.

When making this decision you are also going to need to take into account your overall level of discipline as well as your overall level of health. For example, if you feel as though you have a lot of weight to lose, starting with something less extreme than intermittent fasting might be a better choice until you are already moving in the right direction. Starting off with a diet plan that has such a high learning curve can be detrimental to your weight loss goals if you fail to live up to the strict regulations early on. Failing in this fragile state could actually set you back in terms of overall progress and make it harder to continue pushing forward in the long run.

Be in touch with your body: While it is normal to experience negative side effects when your body is first adapting to new eating patterns, it is still important to take what your body is telling you into account to ensure you don't accidentally do more harm than good in the process. This is true during the first month of intermittent fasting when you are more likely to feel irritable, angry, weak, faint, lightheaded or shaky.

While it is likely that you will experience some of these symptoms to one degree or another, it is important to not push yourself too far, too fast and if any of them become too much and instead give your body a rest before continuing. Maintaining your overall health is a crucial part of successfully fasting intermittently in the long turn and pushing yourself to the verge of literally passing out from hunger is never a good idea, regardless of the circumstances.

Keep your expectations measurable: While the first month or two of your intermittent fasting plan will likely come with larger than average weight loss totals, you are going to need to keep in mind that they are going to taper off once your body gets used to the new eating pattern. Instead of trying to starve yourself in order to keep it up, it is important to instead become used to the fact that any diet should only result in between 1 and 2 pounds of healthy weight loss per week. Anything more than that is simply unhealthy.

Furthermore, you will want to keep in mind that any form of dieting is also going to come with weight loss plateaus where you likely won't lose anything for a week or two at a time. It is important to stay the course when this occurs as opposed to making radical changes to your diet based on a temporary loss of effectiveness. Failing to stay the course in this scenario is only going to lead to scenarios where your body shuts down all weight loss out of confusion for what exactly is going on. Slow and steady will win the race every time, stay the course and your weight loss will always get back on track eventually.

If your weight loss plateaus for 3 weeks or more, then a diet reset is the best solution for both your physical and mental health. During this period you should stick to your IF protocol and fast at the same time, but you can be more relaxed on your food choices during your eating periods. While this may seem counter-intuitive in the short-term, it has innumerable long term benefits. Diet resets should be taken at least twice a year for a 1 week period.

Don't make excuses: While it is important to not try intermittent fasting for the first time when your schedule is extremely busy, it is also important to not use minor reasons for not getting started keep popping up time and again. If this is the case then these reasons are more likely to be thinly-veiled excuses and the longer you abide by them the more difficult it will be to actually get started fasting.

Eventually, you are just going to need to tell yourself that enough is enough and get down to the business of doing your first intermittent fast. Remember, the only person who can motivate you to stick with it in the long run is you. This is why it is so important to not let yourself down and commit to finding the success that can be achieved by finally succeeding when it comes to the weight loss goals of your dreams.

Ensure your goals are realistic: Once you have managed to start using an intermittent fasting meal plan effectively, it is important that you don't expect too much from the plan too soon. Most importantly, 3,500 calories is a pound of fat but that type of loss doesn't take muscle building into account meaning that if you are exercising at the same time it is only logical that sometimes your weekly total is going to be less than it otherwise would be. This will happen despite the fact that you are feeling and looking better than you did before.

If you find yourself feeling discouraged when it comes to a presumed lack of results, you should take a moment and consider how long it took you to get to the point you are at now. With that amount of time in mind, you will then want to ask yourself why you would possibly expect to be able to reach your goals in less time than it took for you to gain the excess weight in the first place. Keeping a realistic perspective on the situation will make it much easier to follow through during the early days and thus, more effectively turn your new way of eating into a lifelong habit.

Take it slow: If you have never gone more than 12 hours without eating prior to your first day of intermittent fasting then you are most likely going to be better off starting at the 12-14 hour point and working your way up from there. Starting with a more extreme form of intermittent fasting is akin to going from 0 to 60 without going through the intervening gears required to get there without burning out. Remember, there is no time frame when it comes to intermittent fasting, simply stick with whatever works for you.

Conclusion

You have learned many things about intermittent fasting and how to use this technique to lose weight and to gain muscle. You have sample meal schedules that you can use to help to get you on the path to health and to a better self-image.

You may want to read this material one or two more times, and make some choices as to what your goals will be. Do you want to lose a lot of weight? Do you want a combination of weight loss while being able to retain your muscle mass?

Next, decide how you will go about reaching those goals. Schedule in the times of exercise, and determine the schedule you will use to eat and what food you will eat.

Then write out meal plans, and make a grocery list of the ingredients you will need to make the first week's planned meals. You may even re-use that grocery list and the ones you make out in the following weeks until you memorize the various recipes to meals you will want to eat repeatedly in the future.

Buy the food you will eat during your first week, and be sure to get rid of any junk food and extra carbohydrate food that is in your kitchen. Make your first meal according to the plan you worked out for yourself. Cook the next meal. Take it one meal and one day at a time until you have formulated healthy habits and your body starts to crave "real" food and exercise.

Finally, if you found this book useful, I would greatly appreciate it if you would review this book on Amazon.

Thank you for reading.

-This page is left blank intentionally-

www.ingramcontent.com/pod-product-compliance
Lightning Source LLC
Chambersburg PA
CBHW070817240726
48654CB00007B/383